FOUR-HANDED DENTISTRY

A Handbook of Clinical Application and Ergonomic Concepts

Betty Ladley Finkbeiner

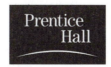

Prentice
Hall

Upper Saddle River, New Jersey 07458

Library of Congress Cataloging-in-Publication Data
Finkbeiner, Betty Ladley, 1939–
  Four-handed dentistry : a handbook of clinical application
and ergonomic concepts / by Betty Ladley Finkbeiner.-- 1st ed.
    p. ; cm.
  Includes bibliographical references and index.
  ISBN 0-13-030413-1
    1. Dentistry--Handbooks, manuals, etc. 2. Human
engineering--Handbooks, manuals, etc. 3. Dental offices--
Design--Handbooks, manuals, etc. I. Title.
    [DNLM: 1. Dentistry--methods. 2. Dental Assistants--
utilization. 3. Efficiency. 4. Human Engineering. 5. Patient
Care Team. 6. Task Performance and Analysis. WU 100
F499f2001]
RK56.F56 2001
617.6--dc21
                                          00-057110

Publisher: Julie Alexander
Executive Editor: Greg Vis
Acquisitions Editor: Mark Cohen
Editorial Assistant: Melissa Kerian
**Director of Manufacturing
  and Production:** Bruce Johnson
Managing Editor: Patrick Walsh
Production Editor: Lea Baranowski,
  Carlisle Communications
Production Liaison: Cathy O'Connell
Manufacturing Manager: Ilene Sanford
Director of Marketing: Leslie Cavaliere
Marketing Coordinator: Cindy Frederick
Creative Director: Marianne Frasco
Cover Design: Bruce Kenselaar
Composition: Carlisle Communications
Printing and Binding: RR Donnelly & Sons, Harrisonburg

Prentice-Hall International (UK) Limited, *London*
Prentice-Hall of Australia Pty. Limited, *Sydney*
Prentice-Hall Canada Inc., *Toronto*
Prentice-Hall Hispanoamericana, S.A., *Mexico*
Prentice-Hall of India Private Limited, *New Delhi*
Prentice-Hall of Japan, Inc., *Tokyo*
Prentice-Hall Singapore Pte. Ltd.
Editora Prentice-Hall do Brasil, Ltda., *Rio de Janeiro*

Notice: The authors and the publisher of this volume have taken care that the information and technical recommendations contained herein are based on research and expert consultation, and are accurate and compatible with the standards generally accepted at the time of publication. Nevertheless, as new information becomes available, changes in clinical and technical practices become necessary. The reader is advised to carefully consult manufacturers' instructions and information material for all supplies and equipment before use, and to consult with a health-care professional as necessary. This advice is especially important when using new supplies or equipment for clinical purposes. The authors and publisher disclaim all responsibility for any liability, loss, injury, or damage incurred as a consequence, directly or indirectly, of the use and application of any of the contents of this volume.

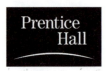

10 9 8 7 6 5 4 3 2
ISBN 0-13-030413-1

This book is dedicated to the six "Js" in my life.

The late Joseph Ellis, DDS, my first employer
The late James Bush, DDS, Professor of Dentistry at the University of Michigan
Joseph Chasteen, DDS, Associate Professor, Department of Oral Medicine, University of
Washington, School of Dentistry
Jim Wells, President of Health Science Products, Birmingham, AL
John Fleszar, DDS, private practitioner, Ann Arbor, MI
Jed Jacobson, Assistant Dean for Community Outreach Programs, University of Michigan,
School of Dentistry

The first taught me caring, patience, and self-worth.
The second believed in me as an educator.
The third taught me organization.
The fourth taught me perseverance.
The fifth has been a caring friend and avid community supporter.
The sixth taught me never to lose sight of my belief in standards regardless of the challenge.

Welcome to the Reader

The clinical dynamics of four-handed dentistry is an ergonomic chairside concept performed by a well-trained dental team in an organized manner. This concept provides a synergistic approach to dental practice that ensures far greater production than two persons working individually in an unorganized manner.

Four-handed dentistry is not a new concept but became inherent in the 1960s to overcome a manpower shortage. Demands were made on the dental profession to provide more services to more people due to the creation of third-party payment. From this time until the 1980s, dental schools taught dental students to work with dental assistants in clinics supported by federal monies provided through Dental Auxiliary Utilization (DAU) grants. Eventually, the grants were phased out. As cost containment became a major factor in dental school budgets, the concepts of four-handed dentistry were diminished, and these clinics were closed in many dental schools.

Ergonomics, the study of the physical relationship between people and their environment, has garnered interest as dentists in the 21st century seek to be more productive and decrease stress. To be effective, ergonomics should not just be discussed; it must be practiced. More important is the concept of participatory ergonomics, ergonomics based on participation of all persons involved in a process. The participants in dentistry are all members of the dental health team, whose safety and job performance depend on their ability to use the skills and concepts from the science of ergonomics. The dentist alone should not make decisions about choice and placement of equipment but, rather, should gain input from the dental auxiliaries who will be using this equipment.

Today's generation of dentists is still faced with the need to increase productivity and reduce stress. However, the impact of regulatory agencies, managed care, and quality assurance has placed even greater demands on the practicing dentist to implement efficient clinical practice methods to ensure a safe, comfortable environment for the entire team. Hence, the rebirth of four-handed dentistry.

In this illustrated manual, the reader will learn the basic tenets of four-handed dentistry necessary to implement efficient procedures for a productive, stress-free clinical environment. The manual begins with the selection and placement of equipment to maintain good ergonomic concepts and presents safe, efficient instrument exchange and oral evacuation techniques that can be applied to common clinical procedures.

The author of this manual "grew up" with four-handed dentistry. She studied under a dynamic research team at the University of Alabama and was mentored by the late James B. Bush, DDS, and Joseph Chasteen, DDS, who both served as Directors of the Dental Auxiliary Utilization Program at the University of Michigan. She has team taught the concepts of four-handed dentistry to dental assistants and dental students as well as practicing dentists who have sought to make significant changes in their dental practices.

As a member of a dynamic health care profession, you, the dentist, dental assistant, or dental hygienist are to be congratulated for taking the first step in planning for a productive, stress-free practice environment.

Acknowledgments

I extend special thanks to family and friends for their continued support. To my husband Charles, I extend my greatest appreciation for being so kind and patient through all stages of my writing. To Kathy Weber, my friend and colleague; Tom Weber, Vice President of Cushing Malloy, Ann Arbor, Michigan; Michael Muscari of Health Science Products, Birmingham, Alabama; and Phyllis Grzegorczyk, Dean of Allied Health and Public Service at Washtenaw Community College, Ann Arbor, Michigan. I extend special appreciation for their continued support of my ideas and for their input on this project.

I also express appreciation to Kristina Spague, a former student and colleague who brings a continued breath of youth to my teaching. Thanks to Mary Govoni, of Clinical Dynamics, and Joseph Chasteen, DDS, from the University of Washington School of Dentistry, for reviewing and critiquing the manuscript. Thanks, too, to Lyn Garry and Sue Null for their help with the photos. To the Dental Assisting Class of 2000, I extend my thanks for being so patient with me during the school year.

A special thanks to Linda Stakley, my secretary, who continues to make me look good in all of my word processing efforts and without whom I could not be a professional.

Contents

Basic Tenets of Four-Handed-Dentistry   **1**

Work Simplification   2
    Elimination   *2*
    Combination   *2*
    Rearrangement   *3*
    Simplification   *4*

Principles of Motion Economy   **5**

Classification of Motions   6
Zones of Activity   8
Team Responsibilities During Treatment Procedures   9
    Team   *9*
    Dentist/Operator   *10*
    Clinical Assistant   *10*

Treatment Room Design   **12**

Treatment Areas   12
Access   12
General Guidelines   15

Types of Delivery Systems   **16**

Transthorax Delivery System   16
Split Unit/Cabinet Delivery System   16
Side Delivery System   16
Rear Delivery System   17

Ergonomic Practice Facts   **18**

Equipment Selection   **21**

Seating the Patient and Operating Team   23

Room Preparation and Initial Patient Seating   23
Patient Positioning   23
Operator Positioning   24
Assistant Positioning   25
Suggested Guidelines for Patient and Dental Team Positioning Regarding Specific
    Treatment Sites   26

Instrument Transfer   30

Instrument Grasps   30
Types of Instrument Transfer   32
    Single-Handed Transfer Procedure   *32*
    Hidden-Syringe Transfer   *37*
    Two-Handed Transfer   *40*
    Modifications for Special Instruments or Situations   *40*

Oral Evacuation   49

About the Author   53

References/Sources   53

Basic Tenets of Four-Handed Dentistry

The clinical dynamics of four-handed dentistry are the components of the process of a skilled operator and assistant working together to perform clinical tasks in a safe, stress-free, productive environment. In this manual, the term *operator* refers to a dentist, a hygienist, or another assistant in discussions of advanced or expanded functions.

The formula for success of the four-handed dentistry concept includes the application of ergonomics. *Ergonomics* is the study of the physical relationship between people and their environment. Any dental professional will tell you that sitting at chairside all day is very uncomfortable and may result in low back pain, tendonitis, neuromuscular, or musculoskeletal complications. Before this concept can be practiced, the reader must understand the following *principles of four-handed dentistry:*

- Equipment must be designed to minimize unnecessary motion.
- The operating team and patient are seated comfortably in ergonomically designed equipment (Figure 1).
- The dentist assigns all legally delegable duties to qualified auxiliaries based on the state's guidelines.
- Patient treatment is planned in advance in a logical sequence.
- The patient is placed in supine position (Figure 2).
- Motion economy is practiced.
- Preset trays are utilized (Figure 3).
- Participatory ergonomics are practiced.

From early research, the concepts of four-handed dentistry have been defined in four basic categories: work simplification, motion economy, classification of motion, and zones of activity. This section discusses work simplification.

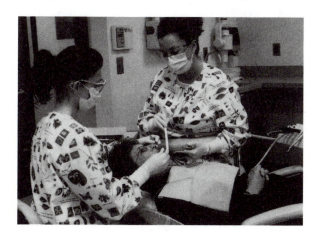

FIG. 1 The operating team and patient are seated comfortably to practice four-handed dentistry.

FIG. 2 The patient is placed in supine position with the head and toes in the same plane.

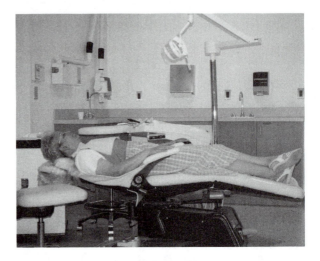

Work Simplification

The concept of work simplification requires the dental team to take a look at the work environment and apply four principles: elimination, combination, rearrangement, and simplification.

Elimination

You can save time and motion if you eliminate items of equipment or instruments while at chairside.

WHAT TO ELIMINATE?

The cuspidor interferes with assistant positioning and inhibits good infection control practice. The bracket tray is positioned in view of the patient and out of reach of the operator. Fixed cabinetry that holds instruments and materials requires extended reaching. Extra instruments that are seldom used take up space on the preset tray and require extra motion to move.

Combination

Nearly 50% of operating time can be saved if you combine the functions of two instruments into one, or two steps in a procedure can become one.

WHAT TO COMBINE?

Use a double-ended instrument instead of a single-ended instrument; use a condenser for more than one task.

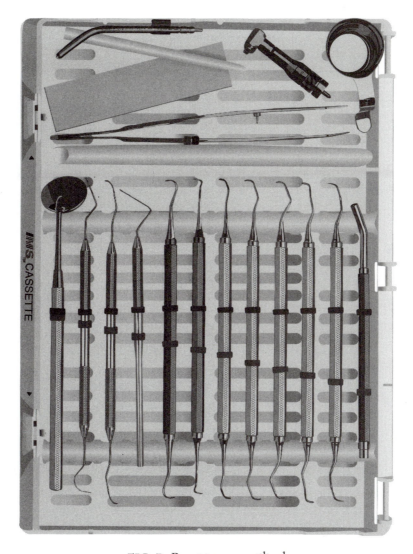

FIG. 3 Preset trays are utilized.

Rearrangement

Consider rearranging instruments on the tray setup to improve efficiency. Relocate equipment that causes excess reaching close to the transfer zone. Review the sequence of a procedure or the scheduling of patients to improve time and motion. Delegate more duties to auxiliaries so that they are productive during a procedure.

FIG. 4 The high velocity evacuator (HVE) tip air/water syringe and handpieces are placed nearest the assistant.

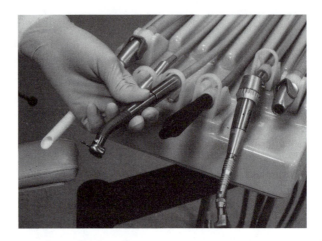

FIG. 5 Back up instruments and supplies can be retrieved easily by the assistant from the mobile cabinet.

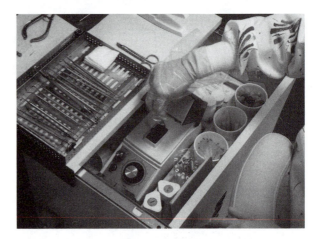

WHAT TO REARRANGE?

Locate the high-velocity evacuator (HVE) tip (Figure 4), air/water syringe, and handpieces on a transthorax dental unit nearest the assistant. Place backup instruments and supplies at the assistant's fingertips in a mobile cabinet instead of on the fixed cabinetry (Figure 5).

Simplification

Make an effort to simplify equipment and procedures in order to function more effectively.

WHAT TO SIMPLIFY?

Consider changing the steps in a procedure to eliminate repetition in instrument transfer. Select multipurpose dental materials to eliminate multiple applications. Delegate bur changes to the assistant.

Principles of Motion Economy

Motion economy refers to the way energy can be conserved and strain on the body reduced by modifying specific motions. This is a major tenet of four-handed dentistry. Each activity in the treatment room should be analyzed to ensure reduction of motion. To minimize or reduce motions at chairside, consider the following suggestions:

Principles of Motion Economy
- Minimize the number of instruments used for a procedure (Figure 6).
- Position the instruments on a preset tray/cassette in the sequence that they will be used.
- Position instruments, materials, and equipment in advance, whenever possible (Figure 6).
- Place the armamentarium on a mobile cabinet as close to the patient as possible (Figure 7).
- Place the patient in a supine position (Figure 8).
- Seat the operating team as close to the patient as possible (Figure 9).

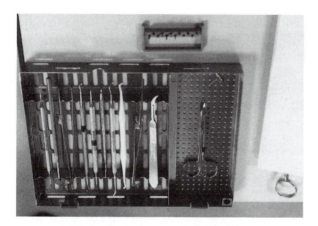

FIG. 6 A minimal number of instruments are placed on the preset tray/cassette.

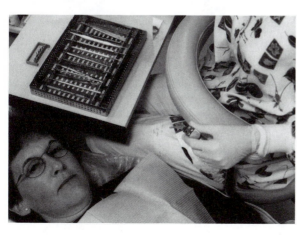

FIG. 7 In advance, the instruments are placed on the preset tray/cassette in sequence of use and positioned as close to the patient as possible.

FIG. 8 The patient is placed in supine position.

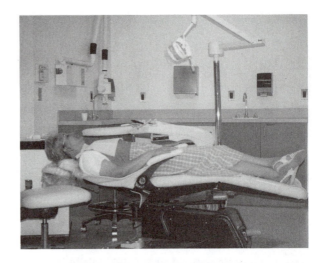

FIG. 9 The operator and assistant are seated as close to the patient as possible.

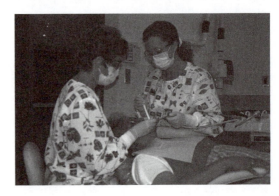

- Use operating stools that promote good posture, and provide back and abdominal support that adjusts vertically and horizontally (Figure 10).
- Provide work areas that are 1 to 2 inches below the elbow (Figure 11).
- Minimize the number of eye movements.
- Reduce the length and number of motions.
- Use smooth continuous motions and avoid distracting zigzag movement.

Classification of Motions

Early researchers classified motion into five categories, according to the length of the motions. As you review these motions, you will note that more energy is expended in Class IV and V motions. Thus, it is recommended that steps be taken to eliminate these motions by rearranging, reorganizing, or planning ahead to ensure that materials and equipment are positioned to maximize motion economy. It may be necessary to reorganize a procedure or rearrange materials to achieve this goal.

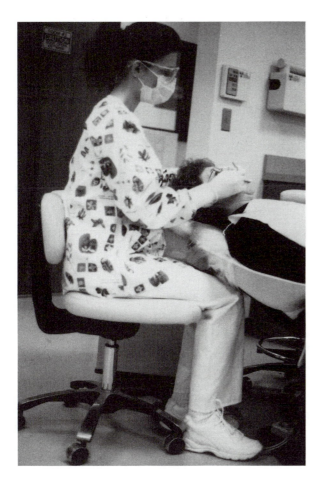

FIG. 10A The operator's stool promotes good posture and provides back support.

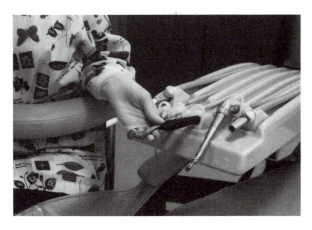

FIG. 10B The abdominal support on the assistant's stool adjusts vertically and horizontally and can be positioned to provide back support.

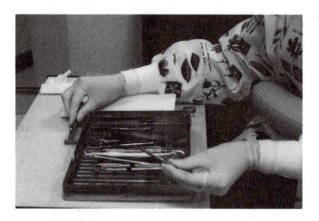

FIG. 11 The assistant's work area should be 1 to 2 inches below the elbow.

The classifications of motion are

- Class I: Movement of the fingers only, as when picking up a cotton roll
- Class II: Fingers and wrist motion, as used when transferring an instrument to the operator
- Class III: Fingers, wrist, and elbow motion, as when reaching for a handpiece
- Class IV: Movement of the entire arm and shoulder, as when reaching into a supply tub or container
- Class V: Movement of the entire torso, as when turning around to reach for equipment from a side or split delivery unit

Zones of Activity

All treatment revolves around the patient's mouth. The area around the mouth is divided into four *zones of activity:* operator's zone, assistant's zone, transfer zone, and static zone. These zones are self-explanatory, except for the static zone, which is the zone of least activity. Instruments that are seldom used, such as the blood pressure equipment, portable curing light, or the assistant's mobile cabinet, can be stored in this area. These zones of activity are best illustrated by using the patient's head as the face of a clock, as shown in Figure 12.

The operator's zone extends from 7 to 12 o'clock, the assistant's zone from 2 to 4 o'clock, the instrument transfer zone from 4 to 7 o'clock, and the static zone from 12 to 2 o'clock. The operator changes position, dependent on the arch and tooth being treated. The assistant seldom moves about in the zone of activity but may find it necessary to raise the operating stool when working on the lower arch.

The left-handed operator's zones are the reverse of the right-handed operator's. The operator's zone is from 12 to 5 o'clock, the assistant's zone is from 8 to 10 o'clock, the transfer zone is from 5 to 8 o'clock, and the static zone is from 10 to 12 o'clock.

Care should be taken by each team member to avoid interfering in the other's zone of activity. Often, an operator is tempted to retrieve an instrument from the tray setup. Such action causes the operator to reach for the item, taking the eyes off the field of operation and

Static zone

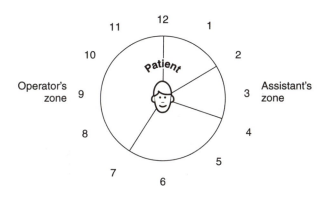

FIG. 12A Zones of activity for a right-handed operator.

Operator's zone

Patient

Assistant's zone

Transfer zone

Static zone

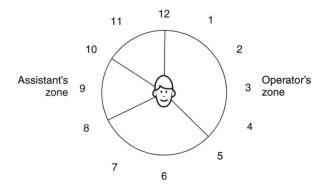

FIG. 12B Zones of activity for a left-handed operator.

Assistant's zone

Operator's zone

Transfer zone

causing unnecessary eye strain. Such activity also interferes with the assistant's domain and can create a disorganized tray setup.

Responsibilities of the team and its members are identified in the following discussion.

Team Responsibilities During Treatment Procedures

Team

General Guidelines
- Be aware of each other's needs.
- Develop a standardized routine for basic dental procedures.

- Recognize the need to reposition the patient and operating team.
- Make changes in positioning as necessary to reduce strain.
- Observe patient movement, especially during syringe or sharp instrument transfer; avoid contacting the patient with an instrument.
- Transfer instruments only within the transfer zone.

Dentist/Operator

General Guidelines
- Develop a nonverbal signal denoting a need to exchange an instrument.
- When necessary, give advance distinct verbal direction to communicate a need for a different instrument or material.

Positioning Guidelines
- Maintain a working position within the operator's zone; avoid legs interfering with the static or assistant's zone.

Transfer Guidelines
- Confine eye focus to the field of operation.
- Confine hand and arm movement to the transfer zone.
- Avoid twisting and turning to reach instruments.
- Exchange instruments only in the transfer zone.
- Avoid removing instruments from the preset tray/cassette.
- Return instruments to the assistant to return to the tray/cassette.
- Rely on the assistant to change burs and transfer needed instruments.

Clinical Assistant

General Guidelines
- Recognize patient needs.
- Recognize any change in procedure.
- Develop a thorough understanding of the procedure.

Positioning Guidelines (Figure 13)
- Be seated as close to the patient as possible; align legs parallel to the long axis of the patient's body.
- Position feet on the stool rim instead of the floor to avoid leaning forward.
- Position the mobile cabinet top over the legs and as close to the chair as possible.

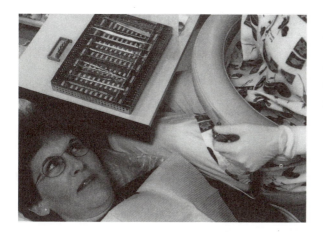

FIG. 13 The assistant is seated as close to the patient as possible; legs parallel to the long axis of the patient's body, with the mobile cabinet extending over the top of the legs, and positioned as close to the patient chair as possible.

Transfer Guidelines
- Anticipate the operator's need.
- When transferring an instrument, position the working end for the proper arch; up for the maxilla and down for the mandible.
- Follow a safe standardized exchange procedure.
- Change burs and maintain handpiece positioning.
- Exchange instruments only in the transfer zone.
- Remove debris from instruments before returning to the tray.
- Maintain instruments and materials in sequence of use.
- Keep the preset tray/cassette and work area free of debris.

Treatment Room Design

Architects, dental suppliers, and equipment manufacturers for years have designed dental treatment rooms. Unfortunately, consideration for the ergonomic concepts of four-handed dentistry and safe practice are not always accomplished. Some manufacturers place great emphasis on patient comfort. This is good. However, primary concern should be for the dental health team's comfort, since they will be working in this environment for many hours each day and the patient is seated for only a short period of time at periodic intervals.

As mentioned in the introduction to this handbook, participatory ergonomics must be practiced to achieve maximum productivity and reduce stress for the entire dental team. Though many dentists may assume primary responsibility for final selection of the equipment, all staff members must be involved in the decision making, since the auxiliaries are an integral part of a successful four-handed dentistry practice. To achieve a safe, ergonomic treatment environment, the following factors must be considered:

Treatment Areas

- Provide a treatment room size that conforms to the guidelines of the Americans with Disabilities Act.
- Create traffic patterns that eliminate congestion and potential for cross contamination.
- Select a transthorax delivery system that places the unit across the patient's thorax area; avoid side and rear delivery systems, since they require increased motion and stress. The transthorax unit promotes safe practice and ergonomic concepts (Figure 14).
- Provide a mobile cabinet that houses major equipment and backup supplies and is free of umbilical attachments (Figure 15).
- Locate all instruments within a 20-inch radius of the assistant's hand for efficient transfer; accessibility to handpieces and other dynamic instrumentation must be primary to the assistant and secondary to the operator. Avoid instrumentation on the assistant's mobile cabinet; it impairs movement and may hamper office cleaning (Figure 16).
- Position handpieces on the dental unit by frequency of use (Figure 17).
- Provide separate sink areas for the assistant and the operator, and include hands-free controls.
- Use minimal fixed cabinetry, only enough to store trays/cassettes and large supportive instruments and materials.
- Provide adequate light to avoid shadows.

Access

- Provide easy access to and exit from treatment room for the patient.

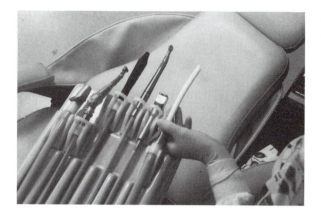

FIG. 14 The transthorax unit promotes safe practice and ergonomic concepts.

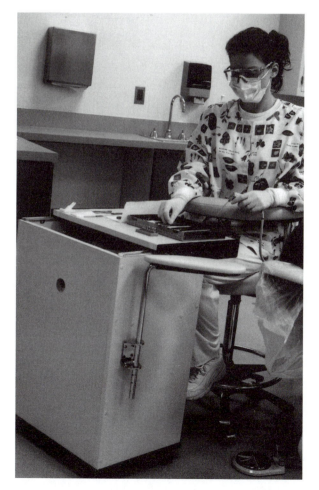

FIG. 15A The mobile cabinet houses major equipment and back up supplies and is free of umbilical attachments. The extended arm rest is provided for the operator to support the non-dominant arm.

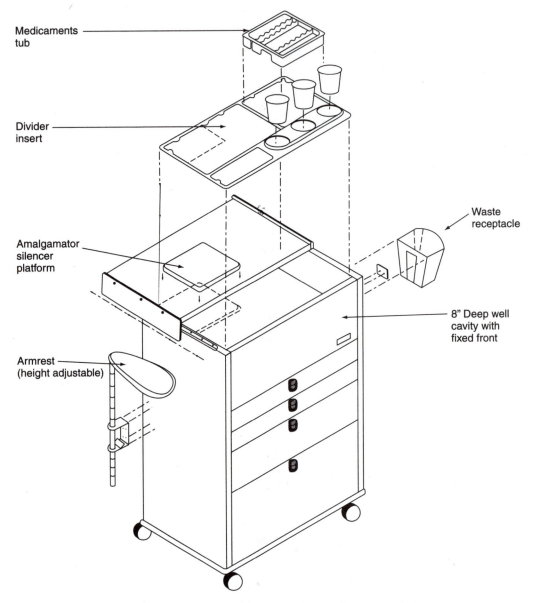

FIG. 15B Schematic of internal components of a mobile cabinet.
Source: Health Science Products, Inc. Birmingham, AL

- Provide a convenient traffic pattern to the treatment support areas such as sterilization, radiography, supply storage, and business office.
- When possible, create a pass-through area that separates clean from nonclean equipment and materials.

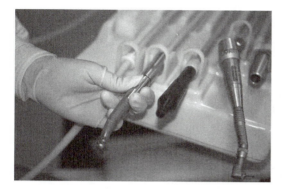

FIG. 16 Instruments on the unit are placed within a 20-inch radius of the assistant's hand for efficient transfer.

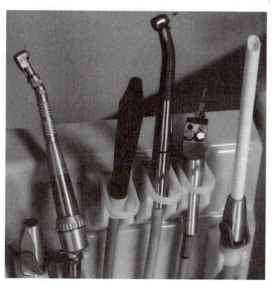

FIG. 17 Handpieces are located on the dental unit by frequency of use.

Assistant's side

General Guidelines

- Provide a location for the patient clinical record area that is free from potential aerosol contamination.
- Provide adequate ventilation.
- Create a warm, comfortable decor, with rounded corners when possible.
- Evaluate the cleanliness of the facility constantly.

Types of Delivery Systems

The basic dental unit delivery systems that have been available over the years include transthorax, side delivery, rear delivery, and split-unit/cabinet delivery. The only system that does not compromise the principles of four-handed dentistry and motion economy is the transthorax system. The following graphics clearly differentiate the application of the time and motion concepts to each of these systems.

Transthorax Delivery System

A transthorax unit (Figure 18A) is positioned across the thorax area of the patient. In other words, it is placed between the neck and the abdomen. For the assistant working with a right-handed operator, all of the instruments are within easy reach of the left hand.

In this system, there are no compromises. The unit is located near the assistant, with the handpieces and other instruments at the fingertips. The dental unit can be moved over the patient within a 20-inch radius of the assistant's hand for efficient transfer. The mobile cabinet provides an adequate work surface that can be moved over the lap of the assistant. There are no connecting umbilical cords to the mobile cabinet, thus making routine cleaning easy.

Split-Unit/Cabinet Delivery System

The split-unit/cabinet delivery system places part of the dental unit on the operator's side with an extended bracket arm (Figure 18B). Some systems include a bracket table near the bracket arm. Other components such as the high-velocity evacuator (HVE) and air/water syringe are placed on the assistant's mobile cabinet. This unit style requires the dentist to grasp the handpieces and compromises instrument transfer between the assistant and the operator. The assistant can only use the HVE and the air/water syringe that are attached to the mobile cabinet and cannot transfer handpieces or change burs. This essentially causes the procedure to stop periodically, thus decreasing productivity. Often, mobile cabinets used in this system are not designed to contain backup instruments and adequate storage for dental materials. The split-unit design compromises the assistant's work area and requires that backup instruments be placed in tubs on fixed cabinetry. This position requires additional motion to retrieve the needed items and opens the door to cross contamination of instruments and materials stored in the tubs or other containers.

Side Delivery System

In the side delivery system, the dental unit is either on a bracket arm attached to the chair or is a separate unit on the operator's side (Figure 18C). This unit does not promote good ergonomic practice.

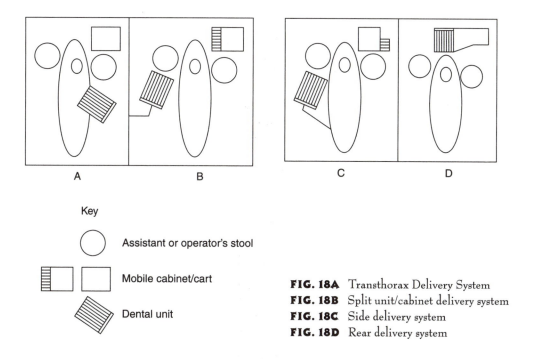

A   B   C   D

Key

○   Assistant or operator's stool

▦ ▢   Mobile cabinet/cart

▨   Dental unit

FIG. 18A Transthorax Delivery System
FIG. 18B Split unit/cabinet delivery system
FIG. 18C Side delivery system
FIG. 18D Rear delivery system

This system requires that the dentist pick up the handpieces. The dentist must remove his or her eyes from the treatment site; twist and turn to grasp the instrument; and then refocus. This results in stress and fatigue. The assistant cannot reach the instruments to exchange handpieces or change burs, thus reducing productivity. Often in this setup, HVE is installed on the assistant's side of the chair, and this pushes the assistant away from the chair. At times, HVE hoses are located on the mobile cabinet. The concern here should be whether the addition of the hoses to this cabinet diminishes the cabinet's effectiveness. It may also require an umbilical cord to the cabinet, resulting in impaired movement and hampering office cleaning. (See key to chart in Figure 18A, B, C, and D.)

Rear Delivery System

In the rear delivery system (Figure 18D), the doctor must pick up the handpieces. It is impossible for the assistant to reach these handpieces without strain. This system requires the doctor to exert severe twisting and turning as well as eyestrain, since the doctor is forced to turn from the operating field to pick up a handpiece. This system severely compromises instrument positioning between the doctor and the assistant, therefore reducing productivity. It also increases pullback on handpiece tubing. As in the previous system, umbilical cords may impair movement and hamper office cleaning.

Ergonomic Practice Facts

Since dentistry is a self-employed profession, little data are available to validate disability patterns that plague the dental health care worker. However, a 1987 survey of 2,000 American Dental Association members found musculoskeletal pain to be an occupational ailment for 60% of general dentists. These dentists reported that they experienced this discomfort from 65 to 125 days each year and that it was the cause for absenteeism, increased breaks, and modifications in the way they perform procedures. The book *Ergonomics and the Dental Care Worker,* (Murphy, 1998) is a reader-friendly reference filled with comprehensive chapters from well-known contributors that offer detailed evaluation of ergonomics including anatomy, physiology, psychology, engineering, design, and management.

Several ergonomic factors surface during equipment design. General factors that should be considered in equipment design include the following:

- Instruments should be easy to use in an ergonomically efficient posture.
- Instruments should be well maintained to ensure that moving parts are well lubricated.
- The force needed to operate and the repetitions needed to produce work from a piece of equipment or instrument should be minimized.
- When possible, a handpiece should be used instead of a manual hand instrument. For instance, grasping a hand-cutting instrument or an endodontic file requires more force to grip the object than using a handpiece.
- Hoses on handpieces and evacuators should be of adequate length to allow the operator to place them into position that maintains an ergonomically sound posture.
- Hoses should be able to be locked into position to prevent pullback on the operator (Figure 19).
- The patient chair must provide support for the patient's entire body in every position (Figure 20).
- The chair back and headrest must combine strength with thinness (Figure 20).
- The patient chair should move automatically whenever possible so that the dental care workers do not have to adjust or lift it.
- Handpieces should rotate and turn with minimal effort.
- Retentive mechanisms for holding a bur in place must allow the assistant to remove and replace the bur easily (Figure 21).
- The diameter of a handpiece should be relatively larger at the base, maintaining a large diameter in the middle, and narrowing quickly at the working end (Figure 22A).
- Switches on handpieces and HVE systems must move with minimal effort. Too much force or repetition of movement may also lead to carpal tunnel syndrome (Figure 22B).
- Knurled or cross-hatched surfaces require less force to grasp than a smooth surface or one with shallow parallel grooves.
- Syringes, such as the air/water, impression, and even anesthetic syringes must be selected to promote reduced stress on the thumb and fingers. Select syringes that will allow the operator or assistant to apply force slowly and as gently as possible, while providing adequate flow.
- Lighting is critical to dentistry. Use fiberoptic high-speed handpieces, mouth mirrors, or additional magnification on personal protective eyewear.

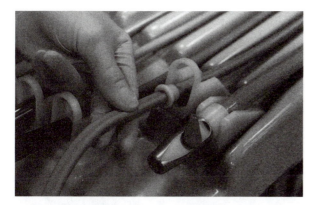

FIG. 19 Hoses should be locked into position prior to transferring to the operator to prevent pullback.

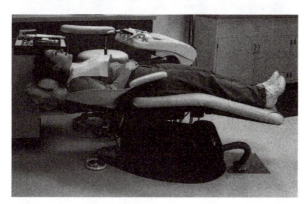

FIG. 20 The patient chair provides stability, must have a thin narrow back, and provide complete body support including arm supports.

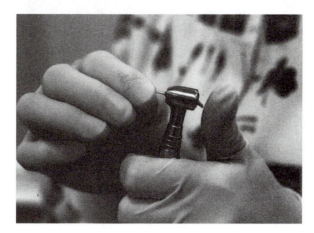

FIG. 21 The assistant can easily change burs when a retentive mechanism is available.

- Personal protective equipment used to reduce the spread of infection must also influence ergonomics. Gowns and caps should fit loosely. Clothing and eyewear must be lightweight, pliable, and as thin as possible. Protective gloves should be sized properly; gloves should be lightweight and extremely pliable. Too small a glove will cause strain and inflammation in the wrist, leading to carpal tunnel syndrome. Hand-specific gloves should be used for long procedures.

FIG. 22A The diameter of a handpiece should be larger at the base, maintain a large diameter in the middle and be narrow at the working end.

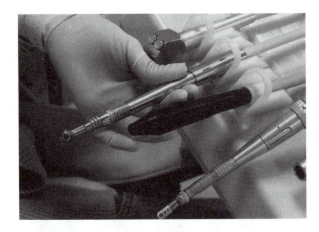

FIG. 22B The switch on this HVE hose moves with minimal effort.

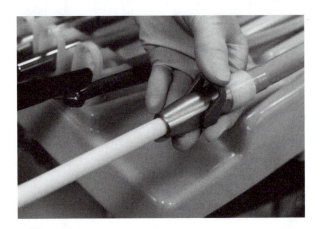

Equipment Selection

Paramount to the success of four-handed dentistry is the type of equipment that the dental team selects. Much equipment is on the market, but often the dental team lacks the knowledge of basic criteria for selecting the equipment. Some of the original research done at the University of Alabama School of Dentistry during the evolution of four-handed dentistry is still among the most sound in meeting these criteria. The dental team cannot successfully practice four-handed dentistry if they must reach for instrumentation, must become entangled in an array of cords, or cannot comfortably reach the patient.

Alan Hedge, Ph.D., Professor, Department of Design and Environmental Analysis, in the College of Human Ecology at Cornell University, notes that the consumer should learn how to judge the ergonomic design of a product. He lists the following suggestions:

1. Does the design of the product make intuitive sense given the goal of the design?

2. Does the product feel comfortable to use?

3. Does the product put the user into a more neutral posture?

4. Can the manufacturer/designer clearly articulate what the ergonomic objectives are for specific design elements? In other words, why is the product designed this way?

5. Does the manufacturer have any research evidence to demonstrate that their product works? How good is the evidence? Is it undertaken by reputable external bodies? What published evidence is there that the product works?

6. Can the manufacturer give contacts for others already using the product?

7. If you are still in doubt and if it is appropriate, is the manufacturer willing to let you have a 30-day trial period using the equipment?*

Use the following checklist to apply selection criteria to the equipment you are using or that you may be considering in office redesign. If you answer "no" to any of these factors, continue your search for dental equipment that meets these criteria.

Source: Hedge, A. (1998). Introduction to ergonomics. In D.C. Murphy, (Ed.), *Ergonomics and the dental health care worker* (p. 22). Washington, DC: American Public Health Association.

Equipment Selection Criteria Form

Patient Chair
- ☐ Does it have a thin narrow back with a concave seat and lower lumbar support?
- ☐ Is it free of wide wings that prohibit the assistant and operator from being seated close to the patient?
- ☐ Does it provide an automatic preset positioner that places the patient in supine position?
- ☐ Is it free of protrusive devices on the back?
- ☐ Does it provide neck and head support for the patient?
- ☐ Can it be positioned for right- or left-handed operators?
- ☐ Is it easily cleanable and free of fabric upholstery?
- ☐ Can it be positioned for easy access?

Dental Unit
- ☐ Is it a transthorax design?
- ☐ Does it adjust vertically and have a horizontal tilt for easy access to operator and assistant?
- ☐ Can it withstand rigorous daily use?
- ☐ Is it designed to contain multiple handpieces and high-tech devices (i.e. electrosurgery unit, automatic scaler) that operate on a single foot control?
- ☐ Is it free of a bracket table and cuspidor?

Dental Unit Components Including Air/Water Syringe, Handpieces, HVE System
- ☐ Do these components contain lightweight, smooth, flexible hosing?
- ☐ Are they easy to use?
- ☐ Does the HVE have a switch that turns on easily?
- ☐ Are there fiberoptic options?
- ☐ Can they be positioned so that the assistant can easily transfer/pass the handpieces to the operator without infringing on the patient?
- ☐ Are the attachments to the hoses sterilizable?
- ☐ Do the handpieces provide a range of speeds and locking mechanisms for hoses to prevent tugback?
- ☐ Does the air/water syringe retain an angled tip that is easily rotated?

Dental Stools
- ☐ Do they provide a stable base with five casters?
- ☐ Do they have well-padded flat or contoured seats?
- ☐ Are they easily adjustable?
- ☐ Does the assistant's stool provide a back and abdominal support that adjusts vertically and horizontally?
- ☐ Does the operator's stool provide vertical and horizontal adjustment with back support?

Mobile Cabinet
- ☐ Is it stable and easy to move?
- ☐ Does it provide easy access to instruments and materials?
- ☐ Is there adequate work surface within 1 to 2 inches of the elbow?
- ☐ Is it free of umbilical cords?
- ☐ Does it provide a movable work surface that can be positioned over the assistant's lap?
- ☐ Does it provide adequate storage with a deep well with space for storage of backup materials and supplies?

Fixed Cabinetry
- ☐ Can it be kept to a minimum?
- ☐ Can it be positioned to provide for maximum floor space?
- ☐ Can it be positioned so the assistant can gain access to backup materials as needed?
- ☐ Is a section of it located far enough away to avoid infectious aerosols coming in contact with records and radiographs?

Foot Control
- ☐ Can it be easily activated with foot pressure?
- ☐ Is it accessible to a right- or left-handed operator?
- ☐ Does it contain a chip blower option?

Operating Light
- ☐ Can it be mounted on the ceiling, wall, or chair base?
- ☐ Is it easily adjustable by operator or assistant?
- ☐ Is it easy to maintain?
- ☐ Is it easy to adjust light intensity?

Room Light
- ☐ Is it easily diffused?
- ☐ Is natural daylight possible?

Sinks
- ☐ Are two sinks available; one each for the operator and assistant?
- ☐ Are the faucets hands-free controlled?
- ☐ Does the sink contain a hands-free soap dispenser?
- ☐ Is an eyewash available nearby?

Seating the Patient and Operating Team

One only needs to walk through the clinics of a dental school to realize that some of the worst patient positioning is learned in dental school. As a student, a dental professional is so involved in meeting requirements that, unless an instructor cautions the student about poor posture, this positioning continues into practice. Each dental professional—the dentist, assistant, and hygienist—needs to routinely assess his or her own position and the position of the patient. If change needs to be made, the procedure should be stopped and modifications made to ensure a stress-free environment. Seating the dental patient and operating team is vitally important to stress reduction and the elimination of musculoskeletal dysfunction.

The treatment room must be prepared before admitting the patient to the area. Suggestions for room preparation and patient and operating team positioning include the following:

Room Preparation and Initial Patient Seating

- Offer to store personal items in a safe location nearby, out of the way of treatment.
- Raise the chair arm for ease of entry.
- Signal the area of the chair in which the patient should be seated by pointing with a hand or providing verbal directions.
- Lower the chair arm.
- Place the patient napkin.
- Offer protective eye wear.

Patient Positioning

The goal of proper patient seating should be to provide patient comfort while maintaining a working position that eliminates stress and strain to the operating team. Some patients such as the young patient, older adult, the pregnant patient, or a patient with congestive heart failure may present difficulty in being placed into a supine position.

Specific guidelines, listed next, should be followed for positioning the patient. Many of these steps can be eliminated if an aseptic chair is used. The aseptic chair enables the assistant to position the patient automatically for treatment in either arch without touching any buttons by hand. This action can take place by the use of the foot control for the chair.

In some illustrations in this text, not all patients may be wearing glasses. Though the Occupational Safety and Health Administration (OSHA) does not require placing glasses on the patient, it is suggested as an adjunct to infection control procedures.

Guidelines for Positioning Patient
- Encourage the patient to move to the uppermost portion of the chair nearest the operator.
- Avoid sudden jerky motions; explain changes in chair positioning to the patient as they occur.
- Raise the chair base about 10 to 12 inches.
- Initially tilt the chair back until the patient's calves are parallel to the floor.
- Place the patient in a supine position, with the knees and nose on the same plane.
- Lower the operating light to a position the assistant can reach when seated.
- Place the unit and mobile cabinet in position.

Operator Positioning

The operator's chair position changes in relation to the area of the mouth being treated. Certain basic guidelines should be followed, however, regardless of the location of the treatment site. These suggested guidelines are listed next.

Guidelines for Patient Positioning (Figure 23)
- The stool is adjusted to allow the operator's feet to rest firmly on the floor and to provide adequate back support. The patient's chair is lowered so that the chair back is nearly in the operator's lap over the thigh area. The operator should be able to move freely in the operator's zone of activity.

FIG. 23 The operator is positioned with feet resting firmly on the floor, back supported, elbows close to the side of the body, shoulders not raised, back straight, and the neck in a neutral position. The patient's head is close to the operator's elbow, and the operator's eyes are about fourteen inches from the patient's mouth.

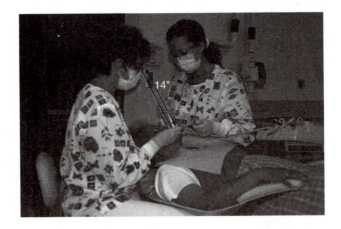

- Use an arm rest attached to the mobile cabinet to reduce arm strain.
- The patient's head is positioned so that the mouth is as close as possible to the operator's elbow.
- Elbows should be close to the side of the body.
- Shoulders should not be raised.
- The back should be straight.
- Keep the neck neutral (straight).
- The distance from the operator's eyes to the patient's mouth should be approximately 14 inches.
- The eyes should remain focused on the treatment site; use telescopic loupes as needed.
- Whenever possible, try to keep the wrist straight.
- Limit exposure to hand-held instruments or handpieces that vibrate.
- Avoid awkward reaching.

Assistant Positioning

The assistant's position, unlike the operator's position, remains relatively the same throughout the procedure, with few exceptions. At times, the assistant may need to raise the stool to improve vision, especially when the operator is working on the mandibular arch. Use the following guidelines for positioning the dental assistant:

Guidelines for Dental Assistant Positioning (Figure 24)
- The stool is positioned as close to the patient's chair as possible.
- The front edge of the stool, or the assistant's knees, are nearly even with the patient's mouth. The thighs are parallel to the side of the patient chair and are parallel to the long axis of the patient's body.
- The torso is centered on the stool.
- The feet rest on the rim of the stool and are parallel to the floor.
- The body support is positioned to come around the left side and to support the assistant's torso when leaning forward:

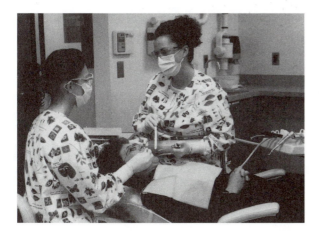

FIG. 24 The assistant is positioned with the torso centered on the stool, close to the patient, the edge of the stool or assistant's knees are even with the patient's mouth; the thighs are parallel to the side of the patient chair and are parallel to the long axis of the patient's body, the body support is positioned to come around the left side and to support the assistant's torso when leaning forward and the eye level is 4 to 6 inches higher than the operator's eye level.

- When seated, the assistant's eye level is 4 to 6 inches higher than the operator's eye level, generally just over the top of the operator's head. The eye level should be slightly higher for working on the mandibular arch.
- Position the mobile cabinet directly in front of the assistant's knees or as close to the chair as possible.
- Extend the working area over the knees or lap, depending on whether the top of the cabinet is forward/backward or side movable.
- Maintain a relatively straight back and neck.
- Avoid forcefully grasping an instrument while flexing the wrist.
- Avoid forceful holding of instruments and hoses.
- Avoid reaching or twisting the torso; position equipment within a 20-inch radius.

Suggested Guidelines for Patient and Dental Team Positioning Regarding Specific Treatment Sites

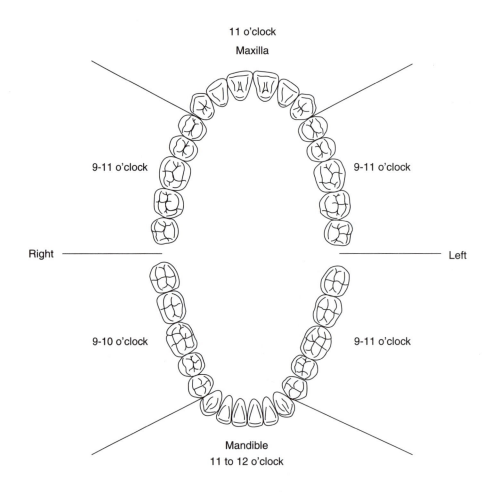

Guidelines for Patient and Dental Team Positioning

Maxillary Right	Maxillary Anterior	Maxillary Left
Posterior		**Posterior**
Buccal Approach	*Labial Approach*	*Buccal approach*
Patient Chair Position—Supine	Patient position—Supine	Patient position—Supine
Patient Head position—Chin elevated and turned toward the dental assistant	Patient Head position—Chin elevated slightly and turned as needed toward the operator	Patient head position—Turned significantly toward the operator with slight elevation of the chin
Evacuator tip- Lingual to tooth being treated	Evacuator tip- Lingual to tooth being treated with half the opening toward the incisal edge	Evacuator tip-Buccal surface, slightly distal to tooth being
Operator position—10–12 o'clock	Operator position—11–12 o'clock	Operator position—10 o'clock
Assistant position—2–4 o'clock, 4–6" higher than operator	Assistant position—2–4 o'clock, 4–6" higher than operator	Assistant position—2–4 o'clock, 4–6" higher than operator
Operator vision—Direct	Operator vision—Direct	Operator vision—Direct
Occlusal Approach	*Incisal Approach*	*Occlusal approach*
Patient Chair Position—Supine	Patient position—Supine	Patient position—supine
Patient Head position—Chin elevated slightly and turned slightly toward the operator	Patient Head position—Chin elevated slightly and turned slightly toward the operator	Patient head position—Turned slightly toward the operator.
Evacuator tip- Lingual to tooth being treated	Evacuator tip- Lingual to tooth being treated with half the opening	Evacuator tip-Buccal surface of the tooth being treated
Operator position—11–12 o'clock	Operator position—11–12 o'clock	Operator position—11 o'clock
Assistant position—2–4 o'clock, 4–6" higher than operator	Assistant position—2–4 o'clock, 4–6" higher than operator	Assistant position—2–4 o'clock, 4–6" higher than operator
Operator vision—Indirect	Operator vision—Direct or Indirect	Operator vision—Indirect
Lingual Approach	*Lingual Approach*	*Lingual approach*
Patient Chair Position—Supine	Patient position—Supine	Patient position-supine
Patient Head position—Chin elevated considerably and turned toward operator.	Patient Head position—Chin elevated slightly and turned slightly toward the operator as needed	Patient head position—Turned slightly toward the operator.
Evacuator tip- Lingual to tooth being treated	Evacuator tip- Labial to tooth being treated with half the opening toward the incisal edge	Evacuator tip-Buccal surface of the tooth being treated
Operator position—9 o'clock	Operator position—11 o'clock	Operator position—9 o'clock
Assistant position—2–4 o'clock, 4–6" higher than operator	Assistant position—2–4 o'clock, 4–6" higher than operator	Assistant position—2–4 o'clock, 4–6" higher than operator
Operator vision—Direct	Operator vision—Indirect	Operator vision—Direct

(continued)

Guidelines for Patient and Dental Team Positioning, *continued*

Mandibular Right	Mandibular Anterior	Mandibular Left
Posterior		**Posterior**
Buccal Approach	*Labial Approach*	*Buccal approach*
Patient Chair Position—Chair back lowered completely, then the back elevated until the patient's oral cavity is at the operator's elbow height	Patient position—Supine	Patient position—Supine
Patient Head position—Turned toward the dental assistant	Patient Head position—Straight or turned slightly toward operator or dental assistant as needed for the site being treated	Patient head position—Turned toward the operator
Evacuator tip- Lingual to tooth being treated	Evacuator tip- Lingual to tooth being treated with half the opening toward the incisal edge	Evacuator tip-Buccal surface, slightly distal to tooth being treated
Operator position—9–10 o'clock	Operator position—11–12 o'clock	Operator position—11 o'clock
Assistant position—2–4 o'clock, 4–6″ higher than operator; raise stool height to improve vision as needed	Assistant position—2–4 o'clock, 4–6″ higher than operator; raise stool height to improve vision as needed	Assistant position—2–4 o'clock, 4–6″ higher than operator; raise stool height to improve vision as needed
Operator vision—Direct	Operator vision—Direct	Operator vision—Direct
Occlusal Approach	*Incisal/Lingual Approaches*	*Occlusal approach*
Patient Chair Position—Chair back lowered completely, then the back elevated until the patient's oral cavity is at the operator's elbow height	Patient position—Chair base completely lowered then the back elevated until the patient's oral cavity is at the operator's elbow height.	Patient position—Supine
Patient Head position—Chin lowered slightly and turned toward the operator	Patient Head position—Straight or turned slightly toward operator or dental assistant as needed for the site being treated	Patient head position—Turned slightly toward the operator.
Evacuator tip- Lingual to tooth being treated	Evacuator tip-Labial to the tooth being treated with half the opening beyond the incisal edge	Evacuator tip-Buccal surface of the tooth being treated
Operator position—9 o'clock	Operator position—11–12 o'clock	Operator position—11 o'clock
Assistant position—2–4 o'clock, 4–6″ higher than operator; raise stool height to improve vision as needed	Assistant position—2–4 o'clock, 4–6″ higher than operator; raise stool height to improve vision as needed	Assistant position—2–4 o'clock, 4–6″ higher than operator; raise stool height to improve vision as needed
Operator vision—Direct	Operator vision—Direct or Indirect	Operator vision—Direct
Lingual Approach		*Lingual approach*
Patient Chair Position Chair base lowered completely then the chair back elevated until the patient's oral cavity is at the operator's elbow height		Patient position-Weat lowered and back of the chair raised slightly so that the oral cavity is at the operator's elbow height

Guidelines for Patient and Dental Team Positioning

Mandibular Right	Mandibular Anterior	Mandibular Left
Posterior		**Posterior**
Lingual Approach		*Lingual approach*
Patient Head position—Chin lowered and head turned all the way toward the operator		Patient head position—Turned slightly toward the dental assistant.
Evacuator tip- Lingual to tooth being treated		Evacuator tip-Parallel to the buccal surface of the tooth being treated with the opening of the tip even with the occlusal surface
Operator position—9 o'clock		Operator position—9 o'clock
Assistant position—2–4 o'clock, 4–6″ higher than operator; raise stool height to improve vision as needed		Assistant position—2–4 o'clock, 4–6″ higher than operator; raise stool height to improve vision as needed
Operator vision—Direct		Operator vision—Direct

Instrument Transfer

Instrument transfer, or exchange, is one of the basic skills of a clinical dental assistant. When an assistant is efficient at this task, the following can be accomplished:

- The operator can maintain vision on the field of operation.
- The operating team saves time and motion.
- Stress and strain on the operating team are reduced.
- When instrument transfer is used in conjunction with the oral evacuator and the air/water syringe, the operative site will always be clean and the next instrument will always be ready for use.

Instrument Grasps

The three most common methods used by an operator to hold an instrument are the pen grasp, modified pen grasp, and palm grasp. A palm–thumb or thumb-to-nose grasp is used commonly by the assistant but less often by the operator.

- The **pen grasp** resembles the position commonly used to hold a pen or pencil and is widely used for most operative instruments (Figure 25).
- The **modified pen grasp** is similar to the pen grasp, except the operator uses the pad of the middle finger on the handle of the instrument. Some operators prefer this method, since they feel it provides more strength and stability in some procedures.
- The **palm grasp** is used for bulky instruments. It is commonly used for surgical forceps, rubber damp clamp forceps, and the air/water syringe (Figure 26).
- The **palm–thumb or thumb-to-nose grasp** is used by the assistant for holding the oral evacuator. The operator may use this with instruments that require a more vertical movement (Figure 27).

FIG. 25 The pen grasp.

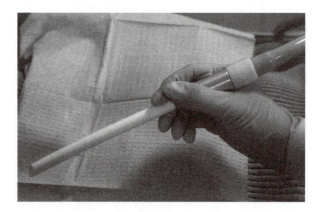

30

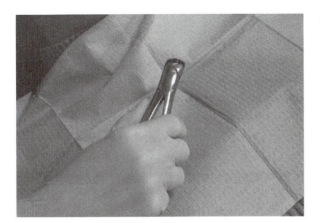

FIG. 26 The palm grasp.

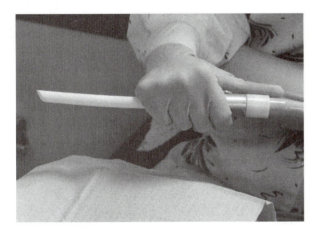

FIG. 27A The thumb-to-nose grasp is used by the assistant for holding the oral evacuator.

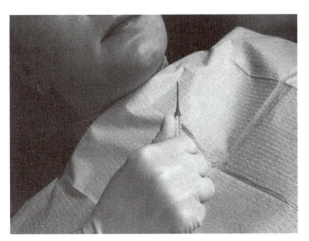

FIG. 27B The palm-thumb grasp is used by the operator with some types of hand instruments.

When using an instrument with the pen or modified pen grasp, the operator must maintain a fulcrum. A fulcrum is the point on a tooth or the nearby tissue where the operator's hand is stabilized to allow the instrument to be used more comfortably. It ensures safety by preventing slippage of the instrument, which could result in injury to the patient.

Types of Instrument Transfer

There are three basic instrument transfers: single-handed, two-handed, and hidden-syringe transfer. The single-handed transfer is used during most common treatment procedures. The two-handed transfer is used when transferring bulky instruments such as the rubber dam clamp forceps or surgical forceps. The hidden-syringe transfer, which also occurs within the transfer zone, enables the operator to receive the anesthetic syringe out of the vision of the patient and thus reduces patient stress.

Single-Handed Transfer Procedure (for Right-Handed Operator)

The single-handed transfer procedure requires that the assistant transfer instruments with the left hand and hold the oral evacuator tip and air/water syringe in the right hand (Figure 28). When working with a left-handed operator, all the positions are reversed.

The assistant's hand is divided into two parts, the pick up and the delivery portions (Figure 29A). For practical understanding, the following discussion defines the fingers of the hand as the thumb, first, second, third, and fourth (the small finger) (Figure 29B). Though some assistants receive the used instrument with only the small finger, you will find that the use of the small and third finger provide more stability.

Some assistants are tempted to flip or twirl the instrument back into the delivery portion of the hand. This can pose danger to the patient if the instrument suddenly flips out of the hand. When the used instrument is received back from the operator in the pick up portion of the hand, the assistant should roll the instrument with the thumb back to the delivery portion of the hand.

FIG. 28 When transferring instruments with a single handed transfer to a right-handed operator the assistant transfers instruments with the left hand and holds the oral evacuator tip and air/water syringe in the right hand.

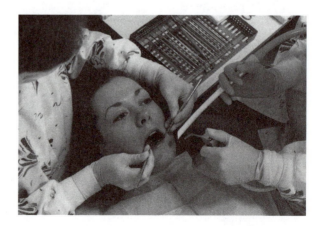

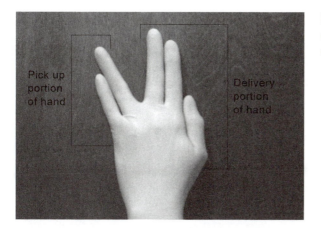

FIG. 29A The assistant's transfer hand is divided into two parts, the pick up and the delivery portion.

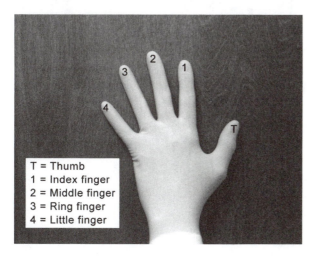

FIG. 29B The fingers of the assistant's transfer hand include the thumb, first, second, third and fourth (the small finger).

The step-by-step procedure for instrument transfer is described next.

INSTRUMENT TRANSFER PROCEDURE OUTLINE

Preparation (Figure 30)

- Assemble instruments in sequence of use.
- Place the instrument trays as close to the patient as possible.
- Place auxiliary equipment such as anesthesia or rubber dams on the mobile cabinet farthest from the patient.
- Pick up the instrument with the thumb and first finger at the nonworking third of the instrument. Rest the instrument on the middle finger, making certain that the working end is positioned for the correct arch.
- At the beginning of the procedure, simultaneously pass the mirror with the right hand and the explorer with the left hand.

FIG. 30A Prior to instrument transfer the instruments are assembled in sequence of use on the tray, the tray placed close to the patient, with auxilary equipment placed nearby on the mobile cabinet.

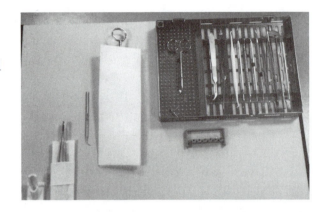

FIG. 30B The instrument is picked up with the thumb and first finger at the non-working third of the instrument.

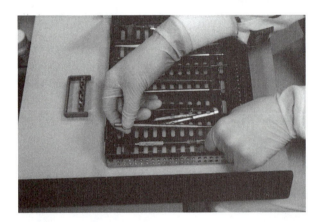

FIG. 30C Rest the instrument on the middle finger, making certain that the working end is positioned for the correct arch.

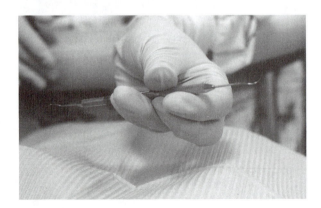

Instrument Transfer (Figure 31)
- The operator signals for an exchange by moving the instrument being used from the tooth and bringing it outside the mouth. When possible, a fulcrum may be maintained.
- The assistant grasps and tucks the used instrument toward the wrist with the pick up portion of the hand.

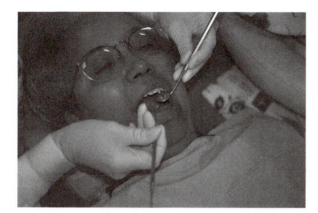

FIG. 31A When the operator signals for an exchange, move the new instrument into position.

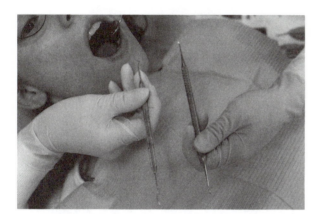

FIG. 31B Parallel the new instrument with the operator's instrument to be exchanged.

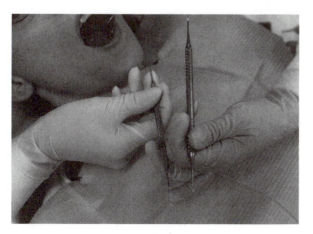

FIG. 31C Grasp the used instrument and tuck it toward the wrist with the pick up portion of the hand.

FIG. 31D   Deliver the new instrument firmly into the operator's hand with the delivery portion of the hand.

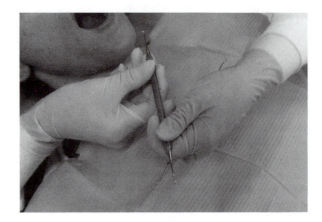

FIG. 31E   With the thumb roll the used instrument from the palm back into the delivery portion of the hand.

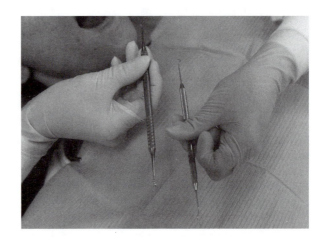

FIG. 31F   Retain the instrument in the delivery portion of the hand if it is to be used again. If not, return it to the proper location on the tray.

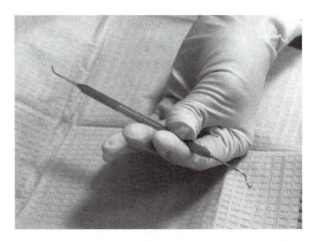

- The new instrument is delivered into the operator's hand with the delivery portion of the hand.
- The operator returns to the mouth with the new instrument.
- With the thumb, the assistant rolls the instrument from the palm up to the ring finger until it is above the first knuckle. Take care to avoid puncturing the gloves.
- Fold the index and middle fingers under the handle, and return the instrument to the holding position.
- If the instrument is not to be used again, it can be returned to the proper position on the tray.
- When the air/water syringe and the oral evacuator are used, the assistant places the air/water syringe in the right hand to free the other for the instrument transfer.

Hidden-Syringe Transfer (Figure 32)

- The hidden-syringe transfer requires the assistant and operator to plan in advance the technique to avoid the potential of a needle-stick.
- A 2 × 2 gauze is passed to dry the site.
- Topical anesthetic may be applied with a cotton-tipped applicator.
- The protective cap on the needle is loosened slightly.
- The syringe is placed in the assistant's right hand when assisting a right-handed operator.
- The assistant stabilizes the operator's hand.
- The syringe is passed to enable the operator to grasp a thumb ring or rest.
- The assistant's hand slowly removes the protective cover. The cover is placed into the recapping device.
- The injection is made by the operator.
- A gauze sponge is exchanged for the syringe. The assistant must be certain to grasp under the barrel of the syringe to avoid contacting the contaminated needle.
- The syringe is placed in a recapping device.
- The mouth may be rinsed at this time if any anesthetic was dropped on the tongue.
- Transferring the syringe in the transfer zone avoids any potential accidents that could occur if the syringe is passed behind the patient.

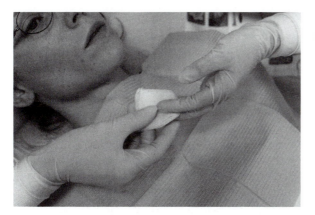

FIG. 32A A 2 × 2 gauze is passed to dry the site.

FIG. 32B A cotton tipped applicator for placing topical anesthetic may be exchanged for the 2 × 2 gauze.

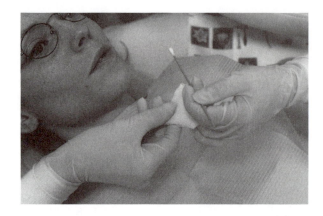

FIG. 32C Stabilize the operator's hand and place the syringe into the operator's hand with the thumb ring securely in place.

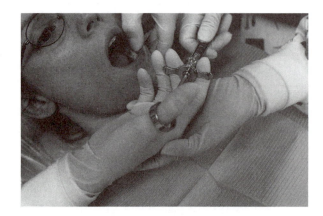

FIG. 32D Remove the protective cover and place the cover in the recapping device.

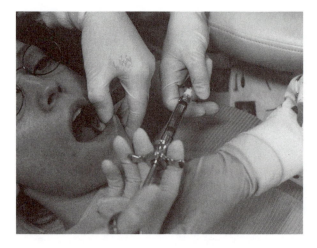

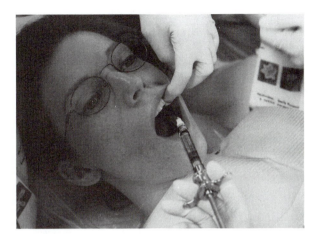

FIG. 32E The injection is made by the operator.

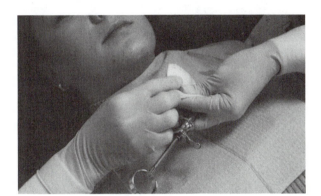

FIG. 32F When the syringe is returned to the assistant be certain to grasp it under the barrel, and transfer a gauze sponge to the operator.

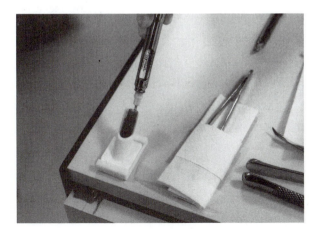

FIG. 32G The syringe is placed in a recapping device and then placed out of the way unless needed again.

FIG. 33A A right-handed operator places the used instrument in the assistant's left hand.

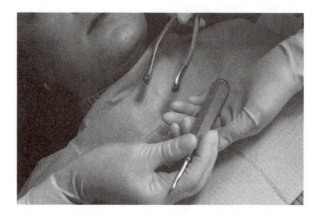

FIG. 33B The new instument is delivered by the assistant with the right hand as the operator uses a palm grasp.

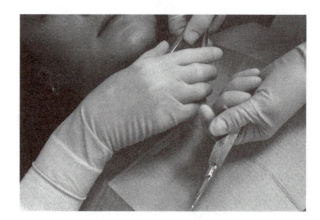

Two-Handed Transfer (Figure 33)

The two-handed transfer requires the assistant to pick up the used instrument with one hand and deliver the new instrument with the opposite hand. This exchange requires more movement and limits the use of the high-velocity evacuator (HVE) and air/water syringe.

Modifications for Special Instruments or Situations

Some instruments and situations require a modification of the procedure outlined previously. The following suggestions may aid during these times:

Dental Mirror and Explorer (Figure 34)
- The dental mirror and explorer are transferred simultaneously at the beginning of most dental procedures.
- Pick up the mirror from the handle end with the right hand, and pick up the explorer with the left hand at the third nearest the assistant.

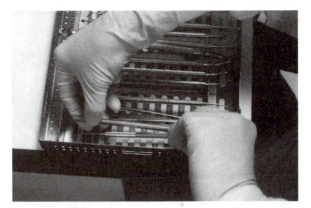

FIG. 34A For a right-handed operator, the assistant picks up the mirror from the handle end and the explorer is picked up with the left hand at the end nearest the assistant.

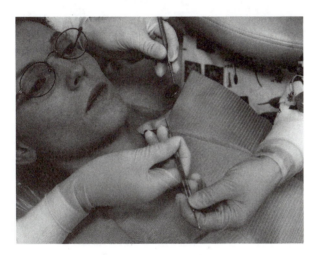

FIG. 34B The two instruments are transferred simultaneously at the beginning of the procedure.

- Position the instruments in the delivery portion of the hands, and when the operator signals, pass the mirror to the operator's left hand and explorer to the right hand in the same manner as described in the preceding section.
- The mirror can be retrieved with the right hand at the conclusion of procedure.

Nonlocking Tissue Forceps (Figure 35)
- The material, such as a cotton pellet, is inserted into the cotton forceps/pliers by grasping the nonworking end of the forceps. If nonlocking forceps are used, the assistant must maintain a grasp on the forceps to ensure the beaks do not separate during transfer.
- The forceps are paralleled with the used instrument that is to be exchanged.
- The instrument is exchanged.
- When the forceps are returned to the assistant, the working end of the forceps is grasped in the palm of the hand to eliminate dropping the contents.

- The forceps are not rolled back into position; rather, the assistant discards the materials from the forceps and returns the instrument to the tray.
- If the forceps are used to retrieve medicaments from a closed bottle, a new forceps must be used for the second application to avoid contamination of the bottle contents.

Small Items (Figure 36)
- For small items such as cavity medication, the assistant passes the insertion instrument to the operator and holds the disposable mixing pad in the transfer zone for easy access.
- A gauze sponge can be passed to the operator as any other instrument.

FIG. 35A When using non-locking forceps, the material is placed into the forceps, with a firm grasp on the forceps, the forceps are paralleled with the used instrument that is to be exchanged.

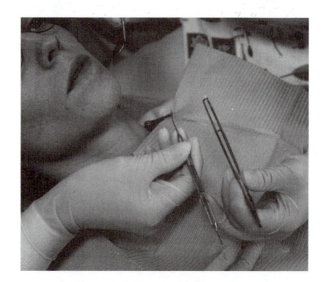

FIG. 35B The used instrument is retrieved while still grasping the forceps.

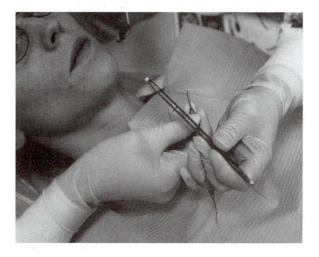

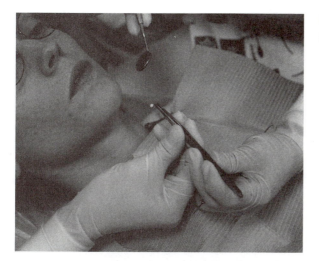

FIG. 35C The used instrument is tucked into the palm of the hand.

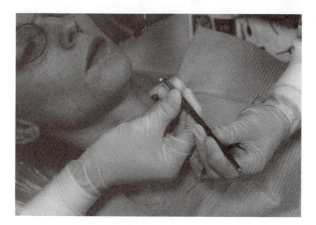

FIG. 35D The forceps are delivered.

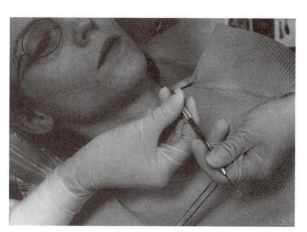

FIG. 35E When retrieved, the forceps are grasped by the working end and tucked into the palm, and the new instrument is delivered.

FIG. 36A Small items such as medicaments can be placed in the transfer zone so the operator can easily obtain them.

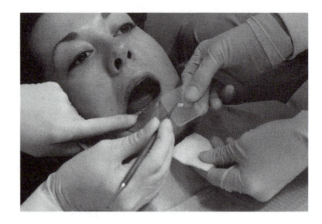

FIG. 36B Small items such as a gauze 2 × 2 is passed in the transfer zone.

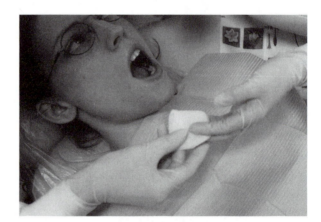

Scissors (Figure 37)
- The assistant picks up the scissors with the left hand, opens the handles slightly, and parallels the scissors with the instrument to be exchanged.
- The operator modifies the hand position by placing the thumb and first or second finger into the rings of the handle.
- The scissors are returned with the beaks pointing toward the assistant.
- The normal exchange then resumes.

Handpieces (Figure 38)
- Bulky instruments can be transferred in the same single-handed exchange as described earlier.
- Be certain the handpiece is free of tension before handing it to the operator to avoid tugback.

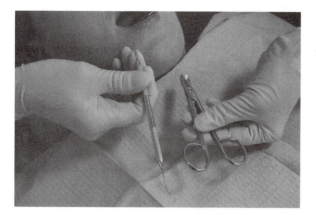

FIG. 37A When transferring scissors, open the beaks and parallel with the instrument to be exchanged.

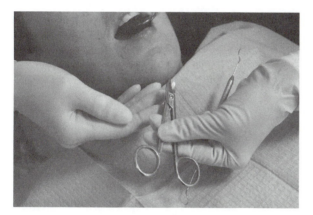

FIG. 37B Grasp and tuck the used instrument.

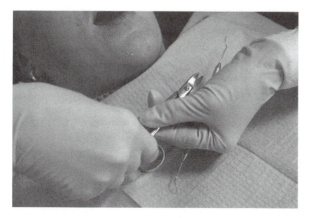

FIG. 37C The operator adjusts the hand to easily place fingers into the handle openings.

FIG. 37D The used instrument is returned to the delivery portion of the assistant's hand and the operator prepares to use the new instrument.

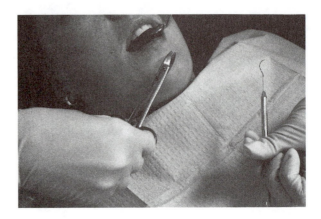

FIG. 38A A handpiece is picked up at the non-working third of the handle.

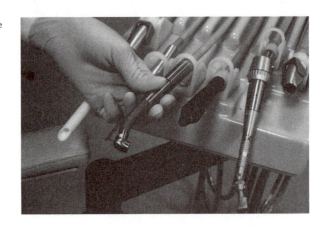

FIG. 38B Parallel the handpiece with the instrument to be exchanged.

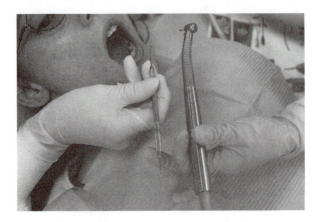

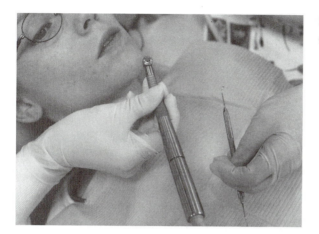

FIG. 38C Deliver the handpiece as any other hand instrument.

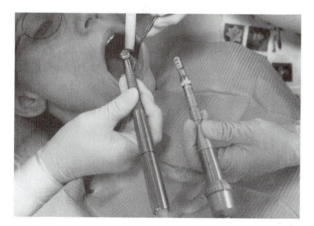

FIG. 38D When exchanging one handpiece for another, the handpieces are made parallel just as when exchanging small hand instruments.

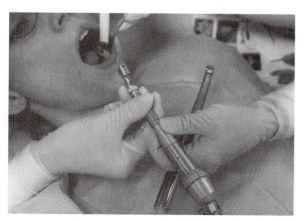

FIG. 38E The used handpiece is retrieved in the pick up portion of the hand and the new handpiece is delivered.

FIG. 38F The used handpiece is tucked into the palm of the hand and then returned to the delivery portion of the hand if to be used again, or returned to the dental unit.

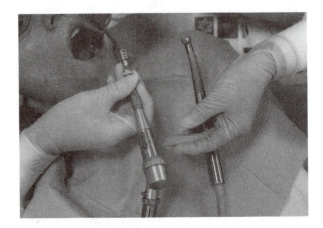

FIG. 38G A reverse transfer is used when the operator wishes to return to the previous handpiece. The assistant picks up the new handpiece with the pickup portion of the hand and receives the used instrument with the delivery portion to avoid hose tangling.

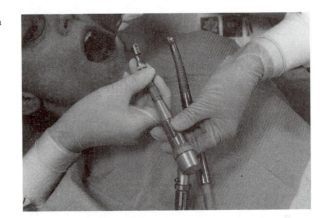

- The return of the handpiece in the pick up portion of the assistant's hand is done in the same manner as another instrument, even though it is bulkier. For this reason, the two fingers used in the pick up method provide greater stability.
- The handpiece is returned to the dental unit.
- When the operator is using a handpiece and wishes to return to the previous hand-piece, the hoses will become tangled in the traditional transfer. The assistant should pick up the new handpiece with the pick up portion of the hand and receive the used instrument with the delivery portion of the hand. This is a bit bulky, but will ensure that the hoses will not become tangled and disrupt the operator's progress.

Oral Evacuation

Since the patient is placed in supine position, it is necessary to provide an efficient system to remove fluids and debris from the oral cavity in a rapid, efficient manner. A high-velocity evacuation system is necessary to accomplish this task. The traditional saliva ejector can act as an adjunct but is not an efficient ergonomic system in four-handed dentistry.

The basic guidelines for oral evacuation follow:

Guidelines for Efficient Oral Evacuation (Figure 39)
- Select the appropriate end of the evacuator tip. Most tips provide a beveled end that may be used in the anterior or posterior areas of the mouth.
- Grasp the tip in a thumb-to-nose or pen grasp. The thumb-to-nose grasp aids in more secure retraction.
- When working with a right-handed operator, the assistant uses the right hand to operate the high-velocity evacuator (HVE) tip and reverses the hand when working with a left-handed operator.
- Place the evacuator tip before the operator places the handpiece and/or mirror.
- Place the tip as close to the tooth as possible.
- Place the edge of the evacuator tip even with or slightly above the occlusal or incisal edge of the tooth.
- Place the tip near the tooth surface closest to the assistant. When working with a right-handed operator on the right side of the mouth, the assistant places the tip on the lingual tooth surface; and on the left side of the mouth, the assistant places the tip on the buccal surface.

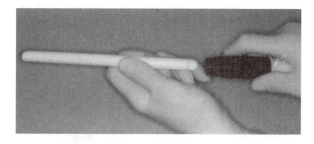

FIG. 39A The HVE tip is placed into the hose for an anterior location. This is shown when the bevel of the tip is not visible.

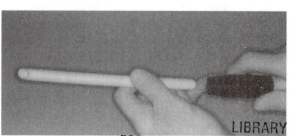

FIG. 39B The HVE tip is placed into the hose for a posterior location. This is shown when the bevel of the tip is visible.

FIG. 39C The HVE hose is held in a thumb-to-nose position for the posterior area or when stronger retraction is needed.

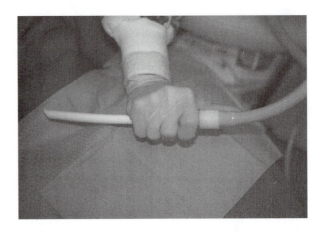

FIG. 39D The HVE hose is held with a pen grasp when in the anterior area or when retraction is not difficult.

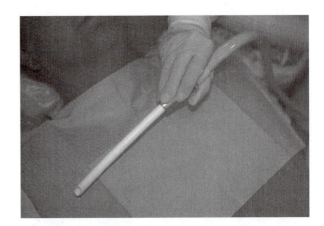

FIG. 39E Place the HVE tip before the handpiece is placed.

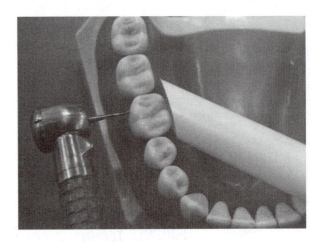

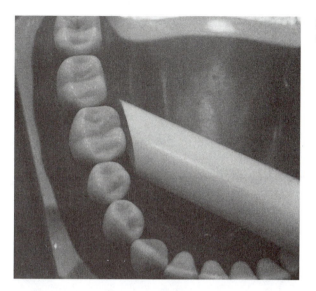

FIG. 39F Place the tip as close to the tooth as possible.

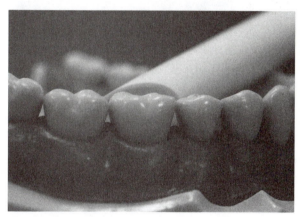

FIG. 39G Place the tip even or slightly above the occlusal surface or incisal edge.

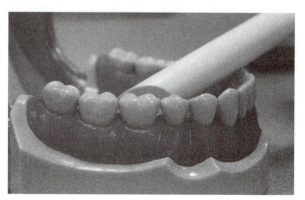

FIG. 39H When working on the right side of the mouth, the tip is placed on the side of the tooth nearest the assistant or the lingual for a right-handed operator.

FIG. 39I When working on the left side of the mouth, the tip is placed on the side of the tooth nearest the assistant or the buccal for a right-handed operator.

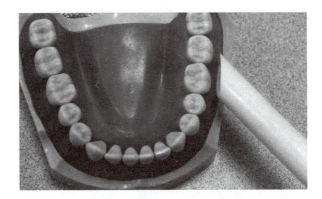

FIG. 39J When the handpiece is placed on the same side as the evacuator tip. move the HVE tip slightly distal.

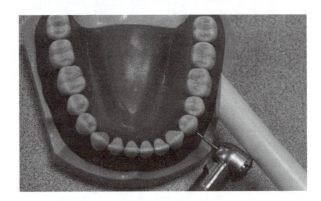

FIG. 39K When the air-water syringe and HVE are both being used during an instrument exchange, transfer the A/W syringe to the right hand and grasp it simultaneously with the HVE hose during the instrument exchange.

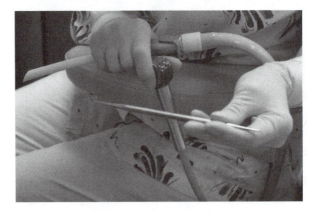

- When the handpiece is being used on the surface nearest the assistant, the HVE tip is placed slightly distal to the surface that is being treated.
- When the tip is used in the right hand, the air/water syringe is used in the left hand until the operator signals for an instrument exchange. During instrument exchange, the HVE tip can be removed from the mouth and the air/water syringe tip is transferred to the right hand, where the free fingers grasp it.

About the Author

Betty Ladley Finkbeiner, CDA, RDA, MS, is a graduate of the University of Michigan School of Education. She is Chairperson of the Dental Assisting Program at Washtenaw Community College in Ann Arbor, Michigan. She has served in this position for three decades. As chairperson of the Dental Assisting Program, she has created a series of on-line dental assistant courses for on-the-job trained dental assistants to obtain professional credentials.

Betty worked in private practice for the late Joseph Ellis, DDS, in Grand Rapids, Michigan, before entering academics. A life member of the ADAA, Betty has served as a consultant and staff representative for the ADA Commission on Dental Accreditation and as a consultant to the Dental Assisting National Board. In 1999, she was appointed by the Governor of Michigan to the Michigan Board of Dentistry.

She has authored articles in professional journals and co-authored several textbooks including *Practice Management for the Dental Team, Comprehensive Dental Assisting: A Clinical Approach,* and *Review of Comprehensive Dental Assisting.* She has co-authored videotape productions, *Medical Emergencies for the Dental Team, Four-Handed Dentistry: An Ergonomic Concept,* and *Infection Control for the Dental Team.*

In addition to her current responsibilities, she provides consulting services to private dental offices in practice management and four-handed dentistry and presents seminars on *Ergonomics in Four-Handed Dentistry* as well as *Fair and Equitable Salary Negotiations for Dental Auxiliaries.*

Phone: (734) 429-4638
Fax: (734) 944-3323
e-mail: blf@wccnet.org

REFERENCES/SOURCES

Bramson, J.B., et al. (1998, February). Evaluating dental office ergonomic risk factors and hazards. *Journal of Dental School Technology, 129*(2), 174–83.

Guay, A. H. (1998, February). Commentary: Ergonomically related disorders in dental practice. *Journal of Dental School Technology, 129*(2), 184–186.

Hedge, A. (1998). Introduction to ergonomics. In D. C. Murphy, *Ergonomics and the dental health care worker.* Washington, DC: American Public Health Association.

Hunk, K. (1996, June). Ergonomics: A case study in preventing repetitive motion injuries. *Journal of Dental School Technology, 13*(5), 35–37.

Liskiewicz, S. T., Kerschbaum, W. E. (1997). Cumulative trauma disorders: an ergonomic approach for prevention. *Journal of Dental Hygiene,* Summer *71*(6), 162–167.

Murphy, D. C. (1998). *Ergonomics and the dental health care worker.* Washington, DC: American Public Health Association.

Robinson, G. E., et al. (1968, September). Four-handed dentistry: The whys and wherefores. *Journal of the American Dental Association, 22*(3), 573–578.

University of Alabama. (1990). Four-handed dentistry manual (6th ed.) Birmingham, AL.

Index

A

Access, to treatment room, 12, 14
Activity, zones of, 8–9
Air/water syringe, 22
Assistant:
    positioning, 25–29
    treatment procedure responsibilities,
        10–11
Assistant's zone, 8–9

B

Buccal approach, 27, 28

C

Cabinets, 22
Chair, patient, 21
Clinical assistant. *See* Assistant
Combination, 2

D

Delivery systems, types of, 16–17
Dental assistant. *See* Assistant
Dental mirror and explorer, transfer of,
    40–41
Dental stools, 22
Dental team. *See* Team positioning; Team
    responsibilities
Dental unit, 22
Dental unit components, 22
Dentist. *See* Operator
Dentistry, four-handed, 1–4

E

Elimination, 2
Equipment:
    and ergonomics, 18–20
    selection of, 21–22
Ergonomics, 1, 18–20
Ergonomics and the Dental Care Worker
    (Murphy), 18
Evacuation, oral, 49–52
Explorer, transfer of, 40–41

F

Fixed cabinetry, 22
Foot control, 22
Forceps, nonlocking, 41–43
Four-handed dentistry, basic tenets of, 1–4

G

Grasps, instrument, 30–32

H

Handpieces, 22, 44, 46–48
Hedge, Alan, 21
Hidden-syringe transfer, 37–39
HVE system, 22

I

Incisal approach, 27, 28
Instrument grasps, 30–32
Instrument transfer, 30
    guidelines, 10, 11
    hidden-syringe, 37–39
    modifications for special instruments or
        situations, 40–48
    single-handed procedure, 32–37
    two-handed, 40
    zone, 8–9

L

Labial approach, 27, 28
Lights, 22
Lingual approach, 27, 28, 29

M

Mandibular anterior, 28–29
Mandibular left posterior, 28–29
Mandibular right posterior, 28–29
Maxillary anterior, 27
Maxillary left posterior, 27
Maxillary right posterior, 27
Mirror, transfer of, 40–41
Mobile cabinet, 22
Modified pen grasp, 30

Motion economy, principles of, 5–11
Motions, classification of, 6, 8
Murphy, D. C., 18

N

Nonlocking tissue forceps, transfer of, 41–43

O

Occlusal approach, 27, 28
Occupational Safety and Health Administration (OSHA), 23
Operating light, 22
Operating team. *See* Team positioning; Team responsibilities
Operator, 1
    positioning, 24–25, 26–29
    treatment procedure responsibilities, 10
Operator's zone, 8–9
Oral evacuation, 49–52

P

Palm grasp, 30
Palm–thumb grasp, 30
Patient chair, 21
Patient seating/positioning, 23–24, 26–29
Pen grasp, 30
Positioning, 10, 23–29

R

Rear delivery system, 17
Rearrangement, 3–4
Right-handed operator, single-handed transfer for, 32–37
Room. *See* Treatment room

S

Scissors, transfer of, 44, 45–46
Seating, patient and operating team, 23–29
Side delivery system, 16–17

Simplification, 2–4
Single-handed transfer procedure, 32–37
Sinks, 22
Small items, transfer of, 42, 44
Special instruments or situations, instrument transfers for, 40–48
Split-unit/cabinet delivery system, 16
Static zone, 8–9
Stools, dental, 22

T

Team positioning, 23–29
Team responsibilities, during treatment procedures, 9–11
Thumb-to-nose grasp, 30
Tissue forceps, nonlocking, 41–43
Transfer, 30
    guidelines, 10, 11
    hidden-syringe, 37–39
    modifications for special instruments or situations, 40–48
    single-handed procedure, 32–37
    two-handed, 40
    zone, 8–9
Transthorax delivery system, 16
Treatment areas, 12
Treatment procedures, team responsibilities during, 9–11
Treatment room:
    design, 12–15
    lights, 22
    preparation, 23
Two-handed transfer, 40

W

Work simplification, 2–4

Z

Zones of activity, 8–9